W. B. HUSTON

Beef Positive

Let animal protein improve your life

This book was professionally typeset on Reedsy.
Find out more at reedsy.com

Contents

First a Disclaimer:

I f you're a fan of double blind, control based medical trials with a sizable number of participants, this book isn't for you.

Who I'm Not

I'm not a medical doctor. I'm not a philosophical doctor. I'm not a research scientist. I'm not even a registered nutritionist (but seeing as how many are nothing but shills for Big Agriculture, why would you read their stuff anyway? They promote that crappy food pyramid).

I'm n=1. **Everything I write about here, I tried. I'm your guinea pig.**

Where I Learned This Stuff

When you're on a journey, you tend to read a lot about the trip. I'm no exception. I'd love to list five or six periodicals as my main sources, but this is the information age. I read books, Substack articles, posts, tweets and watch videos if they capture my curiosity. Those who have graciously shared their info online include in no particular order: Dr. Peter Attia, Dr. Ted Naiman, Dr. Sean Baker, Dr. Casey Means, Rhonda Patrick, Dr. Andrew Huberman, Dr. Paul Saladino, Dr. Gabrielle Lyon, Valter Longo, and many others.

Setting Your Expectations

This book is a small document of the journey I took from being mostly veggie based in my diet to being animal based. Along the way I reduced my body fat, grew muscle, improved my immunity and have managed to look younger than I am. Friends have asked me how I did it, and diet is a large part of my success. For me, health is a journey, not a destination.

There's nothing wrong with having goals. *I want to look shredded for the beach. I want to look good in my wedding dress. I'll show them all at that stupid high school reunion.* Unfortunately, most of us stop our healthy routines once the goal has been reached. And most of us reach those goals by cutting corners and searching for "that one little trick" that will make the process easier.

There is no trick. (I'm looking at you, Ozempic.)

This isn't Disney World where you can pay an exorbitant amount for a "personal guide" to all the rides, who escorts you to the front of the line with no waiting. When it comes to being healthy, you have to stand in line and do your time with everyone else. There are no short cuts. It's just that when it comes to being healthy, most people bail before they get to the ride.

People often conflate being healthy with being skinny, and losing weight. It's not that simple.

Don't jump to conclusions: I am not a fan of body positivity. I don't think being overweight is healthy. And I definitely do not support this recent trend of moving the goal posts in the name of inclusivity so a person's feelings can be spared. Your blood pressure doesn't care about hurting your feelings. Neither does cancer, heart disease, nor stroke.

As a nation we have gotten off track when it comes to healthy goals. We live in a delusion where we pursue losing weight as if it were a recreational sport and yet refuse to do anything that resembles any activity. We need to stop focusing on losing weight and pursue the building and keeping of lean muscle mass. Muscle is the Fountain of Youth. If muscle were a pill, it would be the most prescribed drug in the world.

But this isn't a book about exercise. This isn't a book about building muscle. It's about eating the macronutrient responsible for the creation of muscle.

It's a book to promote protein. Animal protein.

As the saying goes, you can't outrun a bad diet. So whether you're looking to look better or just drop some pounds, the answer is the same. Muscle. And you can't build muscle mass without protein. While you can build muscle with plant-based protein, it is time consuming, technical and would require a large amount of eating. And the fact that most plants come from mono-crop farming practices that have stripped away soil nutrients, vegans and vegetarians are losing out on a healthy diet.

Like veggies, animal based proteins can also come from a mechanized farm where they are nothing but a commodity filled with antibiotics, grains they can't digest and denied rumination. But now there are more alternatives out there for grass fed, free range animal products. These superior specimens make for more nutritious food, but it costs more. However if you compare the money you'd spend on healthy food versus what you'd pay in medical costs, you'd agree that it's much cheaper to go the grass-fed route. And if still you are forced to get your beef from the grocery store, keep in mind that animals are able to convert crappy feed into beneficial food. Steak from Publix still has a wealth of nutrients packed into a small portion.

I'm You

I'm now in my fifties but most people would say that I'm in my early forties. I might even try late thirties if I suggest that I've been in rehab. In other words, I look like a rough thirty-seven or a pretty good forty-five, even though I'm much older. This isn't just aesthetics. I can move easily. I can run up staircases, deep squat for minutes at a time and still hold my own with my teenage kids (but it's getting harder). While all of these feats require cardiovascular and muscular strength, none of the muscles powering me would be able maintain their capacity if it weren't for a protein-centered diet.

But it took me a long time to figure this out.

Call me a product of the times. Where I grew up in the eighties, men with a lot of muscle were muscle heads. And the women—well, there were no overly muscular women except for one. We called her Linda Hamilton. And she didn't show up with arms women lusted after until she did the second Terminator film in the early nineties. I went to a small, college prep high school where excess muscle meant you were dumb. So, wanting to be popular and liked by the ladies, I focused on my wit and long distance running. It kept me trim and helped give me a source of energy that necessitated I be kept far from the caffeine for fear of becoming uncontrollable.

I kept this routine well into my thirties. I would often have friendly arguments with my boss about the superiority of running over strength training. However I was frustrated by how many women I liked seemed to be attracted to all those guys I had termed muscle-heads. I should also be honest and admit that the requirements for being considered a muscle head shifted quite a bit as my lack of success accumulated. Muscle heads in the eighties were the Schwarzenegger want-to-be's who wore tank tops and took steroids. By the nineties muscle heads were simply men who were tall and somewhat muscular. I wanted to have more muscle, but had no idea how to grow them.

By the age of thirty-three, I ran an average of twenty miles a week, usually in preparation for a half-marathon. I was under the delusion that more running would lead to more muscle. So, I decided to train for a full marathon. All of this training fueled by pasta. Lots of pasta. There was some protein, but it was usually chicken breast. I had evolved, after all. Everyone knew that red meat was bad for you, so I was proud that my consumption was reduced to once a month. I also remember the conflict I felt as I noticed that whenever I did eat red meat, usually a steak, I felt good. There was no heartburn. And there was no sleepiness from an energy crash. But I never put together that I might need more protein to be athletic. Long distance runners relied on carb loading. Everyone knew that. So if my diet consisted of three servings of pasta made with American, pesticide-laden wheat for just one of my meals along with a beer or two—I was just being healthy.

When my training for the San Diego Rock and Roll marathon reached mile eighteen, my foot collapsed. I had a case of plantar fasciitis. I was taking Kung Fu at the time (*Crouching Tiger, Hidden Dragon* was big then), and I asked my sifu for help. He was also a personal trainer and was a machine. He had me perform a series of functional exercises like a single leg Romanian deadlift with dumbbells and determined I didn't have enough muscle to run the race. Again, what I heard was I need to spend more time in the gym, not eat more protein.

I spent the next several months building an impressive workout regimen that included over twenty miles of road work, three gym sessions that lasted a couple of hours each and Kung Fu three times a week. And I still ate mostly pasta and salads with some chicken or shrimp. If there was dairy it was skim milk. And the most frustrating thing about all this effort was I looked puffy. I had managed to find a woman who loved me and wanted to get married, but when I got to the honeymoon, I looked skinny and doughy at the same time. No musculature. And given that these were my thirties, I had half given up on growing any extra muscle given that at the time, everyone knew that muscle decreased with age. And while this is partially true, we now know that sarcopenia occurs if you don't work the muscle or continue pursuits to grow it. You can grow muscle well into your seventies. And this should be both a wake up call and source of inspiration to **change our mindset to focus on growing muscle instead of losing fat.**

By the time my daughter was born five years later, my running pursuits had greatly diminished— mainly because I had developed either "athlete-induced asthma" or "seasonal asthma." It depended on whether I was talking to my internist or my new pulmonologist. By this time, I was closing in on forty, and was on a handful of prescription medications like most Americans. What frustrated me was I wasn't fat, so why did I feel so old? Why was I so unhealthy? Why did I need to take these damn pills? Workouts wore me out. There was no visible increase in muscle despite the hours in the gym. I was skinny fat, but I didn't realize that was a detriment. I didn't realize that there were men who were either on the cusp of becoming fat because of how their bodies stored adipose tissue around vital organs before other parts of the body, or there were men who were carrying a large amount of inflammation due to poor diet, like me.

Regardless, due to my diet I was on Prilosec, a proton pump inhibitor (stopped my stomach from making gastric acid), Claritin (for daily allergies) and Advair (for asthma). Advair was a particular milestone in my new growing list of chronic illnesses. A friend of mine who had been in the Special Forces quipped that Advair was known as "the purple disc of death" at the VA given its long list of side effects and the necessity of having to rinse your mouth after every treatment to prevent thrush (a lovely rash that forms on mouth tissue).

Fortunately because of impending middle age, I had made some dramatic changes in my life. I had decided to pursue filmmaking and copywriting instead of remaining in IT. Both of these creative industries are youth centric, so if you want to work, you have to look young and healthy. That drove my pursuit on trying to get in the best physical shape I could. Yes, it's vain. But sometimes vanity can be a good thing. And if you don't think a healthy appearance makes a difference in your career, you're kidding yourself.

The asthma had made it impossible to run long distances outside and I'm not a fan of machines. By the time I started to see a connection between diet and asthma, I had given up running. I guess you can learn to hate anything if you do it for over twenty-five years.

I stumbled upon an online article about Bruce Lee. If you're old enough and have seen some of his martial arts films from the seventies, you know how in shape and ripped he was. Long before Brad Pitt, Lee was about strength, speed, vascularity and an eight pack of abs. Also he wasn't physically huge. He was the perfect role model for my fitness pursuits. It was here that I learned about IF or intermittent fasting. Also at this time, there was an explosion of information on the gut biome and the potential importance of probiotics. Now it could be placebo or who knows, but once I began waiting at least sixteen hours between feeding windows and started taking probiotics daily, my acid reflux went away as did my asthma.

At this point, I was still following the same diet—heavy on the veggies and the grains with some chicken and occasional steak, but contrarian advice was starting to seep in. Once I learned that full fat, grass fed milk was not only not bad for you, but beneficial, I began to question what else was okay that I had once demonized.

Over the next several years, the fasting became longer and more intense and the probiotics became symbiotics (pre and probiotics). The food became less packaged and more whole. Soon I was Paleo and determined to get all processed food out of my diet. It made a big difference. But like many on this journey, Paleo eventually led to Keto. Thanks to the advice of Dr. Peter Attia and others, the concept of sustained energy through a Keto diet became a motivator to become a true convert.

The Keto diet is millennia old and had been used as far back as ancient Greece to treat epilepsy. But like many health movements, the diet of less than fifty grams of carbohydrate gained a lot of traction in the body building community because of how it promoted weight loss while preserving muscle. Dr. Attia gave the diet some sophisticated sheen by pointing out the potential mental health benefits. This helped me forget about its illustrious incarnations from earlier when it was known as *The Scarsdale Diet* or at the turn of this century, *The South Beach Diet.*

At the time, my elderly father was fighting Alzheimer's, and I was desperate to find a way to avoid its genetic wrath. (We now suspect it has little to do with genes and more to do with your metabolism—but that's another book.) Since the Ketogenic diet over time converts the human cells' mitochondria to fat burning from sugar burning, many of the metabolic problems we experience with the Standard American Diet (SAD) are avoided. I went full revolutionary guard with this movement, remaining Keto for over two years. Since the diet requires eating fat to burn fat and deplete the cells of carbohydrate, I was forced to incorporate many animal proteins into my diet. Gone were the onions, peppers and broccoli and incoming were the New York Strips, Chicken thighs with skin and bacon.

It was with this diet that I began to understand the differences between fats. Basically if the fat comes from a seed that needs to be chemically treated, it's filled with trans fats—which have been shown to cause heart disease and cancer (not just a correlation like the argument that red meat causes cancer). These are your Canola, Safflower, Sunflower, Soybean, and Corn oils. Manufacturers will argue that their polyunsaturated fats are a valuable source of Omega 6 fatty acids, but they're not. Their production process of extreme heat and cleansing with industrial solvents makes them radicalized in the bloodstream, negatively affecting tissues. Problem is they are subsidized by Big Agriculture and are in everything from mixes in a box to salad dressings to even being sprayed on certain produce to act as a preservative. Given their high smoke point (the temperature at which a fat breaks down, becomes rancid and radicalized), it's used in all fried foods.

I also realized that saturated fat, if it comes from animal protein is beneficial. This fat has a higher Omega 3 to Omega 6 ratio which leads to less inflammation. It has CLA (Conjugated Linoleic Acid) that may reduce body fat, increase muscle and also reduce inflammation. It contains many essential vitamins like A, D, E and K2—all essential for immunity and necessary bodily functions. Saturated fats from grass fed animals also keep cholesterol in check and add to brain functions and better gut health. It's hardly the bogeyman it has been portrayed by Big Pharma, who are financially motivated to keep people thinking they need statins to help prevent bad cholesterol. (The cholesterol scam is a book in and of itself.)

Then there are the benefits of the monounsaturated fats such as olive oil and avocado oil, but you'd have to be living under a rock not to know about these. (Though there are some scams with these oils as well, covered in another chapter.)

An Embarrassingly Quick and Simplified History

Back in those Paleolithic days, we used to hunt. Most of our nutrients came from the meat of the animals we slaughtered out on the plain. But then Man, with his newly enlarged brain thanks mainly to the fats and proteins he ingested from his primal dinner, tired of the intermittent fasting he experienced between successful hunts and sporadic foraging of berries he might find along the way. He discovered agriculture and soon we were on our way from migrating clans to settlements to small towns to cities to empires with weapons to protect them along the way.

Then a bunch of stuff happened.

And then there was World War II. When the allies learned of the concentration camps, they realized they would need to deal with starvation on a mass scale. Dr. Ancel Keys led the research on fasting and its effects on the human body. His research, especially that concerned with the importance of electrolytes, saved thousands of lives by preventing these victims from suffering cardiac arrest when refeeding due to their potassium, magnesium and sodium deprivations.

When President Eisenhower suffered a heart attack while in the White House, Ancel Keys was once again called upon to research this new epidemic that was plaguing the U.S. Ancel entered into his research with an assumption he wanted to prove. Or an assumption he was paid to prove—depending on your point of view. Ancel was convinced that saturated fat was responsible for the heart attack of the president and all of the other victims across the country. He ventured out to the world to compare and contrast the Standard American Diet to others where there were minimal heart attacks, and then cherry picked the data to prove his hypothesis. His work was the *Seven Countries Study*, where he appeared to prove the negative impact of saturated fat and the benefits of more carbohydrates in the diet. His thesis was controversial because he neglected to include countries where saturated fat was high but heart disease low, like France. It being a government study, it took years to ratify and not until the early seventies had the research's finding (generously subsidized by the sugar industry) been put together in a food pyramid.

Interestingly the invention of the food pyramid and its adoption across the country corresponds to the dramatic increase in metabolic syndrome across the U.S. Moving away from protein and fat, led us away from satiety and toward constant cravings and chronic inflammation.

When R.J. Reynolds realized it was on the losing end of government regulations and state led class action lawsuits due to the epidemic of lung cancer, they did what any other Fortune Five Hundred would do, they merged. They bought Nabisco in the late eighties and immediately put their infamous research scientists to work on processed food. Soon RJR Nabisco was putting out palatable foods that engaged the addiction centers of the brain, making it difficult to move away from sugar-filled box treats to fresh whole foods. Throw in some seed oils, fake colors and other preservatives and you have a crappy food spiral nobody could resist.

Now Big Ag is bigger than ever and has tried to disrupt the animal protein market with vegetable friendly fake meats that are much worse in taste and in health effects than the factory farm variety. Big Ag thought they had the market cornered until they rolled out their Impossible Meat and other Frankenstein proteins. Fortunately they failed to catch on. Now Big Ag is trying to get their return on investment by forcing municipalities to buy these products.

Enter: COVID. Nothing exposed the sickness of our country like this pandemic did. Sunlight. Diet. Exercise. All eschewed for mandated lockdowns, made up distancing, masking that did nothing but show compliance, Netflix bingeing and consumption of shelf-stable highly processed foods. My obsession with spreading what I've learned about a healthy diet came from COVID. Until this illness that shall not be investigated by the same government experts that created it, I was a big believer in Western medicine. But after seeing how corrupt our governing bodies (FDA, NIH, USDA, etc.) are I realized that I was better off finding my own path to a healthy life instead of trusting some institution that could care less. In fact, it's their main profit motive to keep the population sick but alive. It's a vicious spiral battling it out to who will profit more: food companies that produce products that make us metabolically sick or the big pharmaceuticals that produce the medications that treat our new chronic ailments. One thing I know is both hate the small, regenerative farms that are beginning to spring up across the country.

Carnivore vs Keto vs Paleo: We're on the Same Team

We are a tribal animal. We like to be in a clan and on a team. From patriotism because of the country you were raised in, to your favorite SEC football team, to what you eat. We're all searching for community. So, it's no surprise than in this world of social media and hyper politicization, that what you eat is now becoming an expression of your identity. Literally you are now what you eat.

I know, because I'm probably guilty of this. As I previously related, I went from SAD to Paleo to Keto to Carnivore. Whoops. I may have forgotten to mention that last bit. This past New Year, my wife and I celebrated the flipping over of the calendar by foregoing anything but animal protein. It was successful and it's a tool in my belt I will use again, but it's difficult to adhere to unless you have a medical condition you have to beat, it's easy to get swept up in the purity tests that often accompany these diets.

When you choose to go on any exclusion diet like Paleo or Keto or Carnivore, you will run into the purists. They follow a strict set of rules and are quick to inform others that they are not performing as they should. In some cases, the rules are helpful when first starting out. For example, to get into Ketosis, the process wherein the body uses fat for energy by creating ketones for the cells to metabolize, you have to deplete all of your glycogen stores. (Glycogen is sugar stored in the muscle.) And the only way to do this is to reduce the intake of carbohydrates below 50 grams per day. If you're consuming 100 grams of carbohydrate, you're engaging in a low carb diet, but you're not getting into Ketosis (unless you've been ketogenic for several weeks and are engaging in strenuous athletic activity) and you will not gain all the benefits of the diet.

When my wife and I decided to give the Carnivore Diet a try we were bio hacking, not fighting cancer nor MS. (There are now several studies that show a carnivore diet capable of putting people in remission when battling several chronic autoimmune diseases.) We wanted to know if we could achieve some of the benefits others did. If someone afflicted with rheumatoid arthritis could go into complete remission, what could two relatively healthy adults achieve? You could argue it is the ultimate ketogenic diet as your body will be forced to rely on fat for energy but will be able to still produce protein synthesis (build muscle).

The purists insist to be "true carnivore" you can only eat red meat and use salt as a seasoning and drink water. Dr. Sean Baker who coined the term Carnivore Diet when treating his metabolically sick patients disagreed with this approach. He considered the diet an exclusion diet to help people determine what in their everyday diet was making them sick. Everyone's body is unique and what may be ailing me may not be ailing you even if we have the same symptoms. His approach was to be Carnivore until the symptoms subsided and then slowly add back in different foods to find the culprit.

For those on a biohacker's journey, there was no need to exclude other meets like poultry or seafood or even some spices if the body showed no ill effects. But his argument was most people don't remember what it feels like to not have chronic inflammation, so getting everything out of the diet and getting to baseline is important at the beginning. In all honesty, I made it about three days before I started wiggling around the rules and bringing in dairy in the form or Greek yogurt, whey protein powder and cheese. Regardless I was able to achieve Ketosis and enjoy the mental clarity, lack of any inflammation and consistent energy. But we have two teenage kids, and it was winter break and there was no way we could adhere to the diet during a week in South Beach. We gave it a solid try, but in the end the grains got us. We did look great by the way.

While mental clarity and sustained energy are nice to have, the main benefits of getting off the SAD is to heal the gut microbiome. Processed foods wreak havoc with our gut which is where the majority of our immune system works its magic. But it also has serious influence on our brain. It seems that old adage of trusting your gut has truth to it. The Vega nerve connects the gut to the brain as a bidirectional highway. In other words, the brain affects the microbiome, and the microbiome affects the brain. In fact, there are studies showing the connection between certain bacterial strains in the gut and clinical depression, moodiness and addiction. Animal protein provides the nutrients essential to strengthening the lining of the gut as well as providing essential bacteria for gut health.

If you decide to engage in one of these exclusion diets, there are plenty of resources to help online. I would strongly suggest you invest in some electrolyte mixes that don't come in the form of energy drinks and up your intake of salt. These help the body regulate hydration and lethargy sometimes referred to as the Keto Flu.

And if you decide to give carnivore a try, there is one bizarre effect. You will have fewer bowel movements. And there will be less poo. According to Dr. Sean Baker that is because what you excrete is waste; it's indigestible. When on a carnivore diet, because meet is so nutrient dense and beneficial, there is very little that is not digested and metabolized, leading to the dramatic lack of product. When on Carnivore, there's no need to hit the laxatives. You're not clogged up.

It's All in the Blood

Animal proteins are nutrient dense, and each bring with them some unique vitamins and minerals. This is a quick rundown of the most prevalent nutrients to be found in animal proteins.

Vitamin A

It's a fat soluble vitamin. It's stored in fat tissue for later use. Essential for cell growth, a strong immunity, fetal development and vision.

Essential Amino Acids

Amino Acids are building blocks of proteins, hormones and neurotransmitters. Essential amino acids are proteins needed for body functions. Your body can make non-essential amino acids, but can't make the essential ones. Those include: Phenylalanine (for neurotransmitters like dopamine), Valine (muscle growth and regeneration), Threonine (for making skin and connective tissue), Tryptophan (affects sleep, appetite and mood), Methionine (for metabolism), Leucine (for protein synthesis and blood sugar regulation), Isoleucine (for muscle metabolism), Lysine for energy production and immunity), Histidine (for immunity, sex and circadian rhythm).

Vitamin B1 (Thiamin)

It's a water soluble vitamin which means the body can't store it for later use. It must be consumed regularly to aid in energy production, cell functions, including growth and development.

Vitamin B3 (Niacin)

It's a water soluble vitamin used in the conversion of food to energy.

Vitamin B6

It's a water soluble vitamin essential for the creation of red blood cells, neurotransmitters and metabolism.

B12

It's an essential vitamin that has to be consumed and is stored in the liver for aiding in brain activity, creating DNA, producing energy and protecting the nervous system.

BCAA (Branched Chain Amino Acids)

These are three of the nine essential amino acids (Leucine, Isoleucine and Valine) that aid in muscle retention, growth, and exercise recovery. They have to be consumed in the diet.

Calcium

An essential mineral that makes up bones and teeth. It aids in muscle formation, blood clotting and nerve firing.

Carnosine

The only antioxidant found in meat, dairy and eggs.

CLA (Conjugated Linoleic Acid)

It's the most common Omega 6 fatty acid (polyunsaturated or PUFA) found in vegetable oils and naturally in foods. The food based CFA is a trans-fat that might be beneficial for fat loss.

Creatine

It's a substance found in muscle cells that aid in producing energy for intense exercises. Recent studies suggest it may also be beneficial in fighting neurodegenerative diseases like epilepsy and Alzheimer's.

Vitamin E

An antioxidant that aids in reducing heart disease, fatty liver disease, promotes skin health, brain cognition and lung functions.

Iron

An essential mineral responsible for transporting oxygen through the body with red blood cells.

K2

An essential vitamin that may aid in preventing calcium deposits within the arteries while conversely aiding in blood coagulation. It supports the formation of bone and teeth and may even be beneficial in fighting certain forms of cancer.

Omega 3

A fatty acid that aids in the reduction of inflammation as it supports brain and heart health.

Omega 6

It's an essential fatty acid for your diet. The most prevalent form is Linoleic acid.

Phosphorus

It's an essential mineral necessary for bone growth, energy creation and genesis of new cells.

Selenium

It's a mineral you have to consume in your diet. It's necessary in the function of your metabolism, immune system and thyroid.

Zinc

It's an essential nutrient found in your diet that aids in your immune system, cell growth, skin health and may protect against inflammation and acne.

The Best Animal Proteins for Your Diet

BEEF

Beef is a highly versatile protein when it comes to consumption and provides a wealth of variable tastes when cooked. It provides a wealth of vitamins and minerals essential for the building and maintaining of muscle and bone tissue as well as the production of energy. Because of its satiety, it is effective in weight loss as it naturally prevents overeating.

It's a great source of Iron, Zinc, B12, B6, Niacin, Creatine, Carnosine and CLA.

Great for cooking on the grill, stove or oven.

Best cuts for Grilling:

Strip

Sirloin

Flank

T-Bone

Ribeye

Tenderloin

Tri-tip

Porterhouse

Ground Beef

Flat Iron

Skirt

Chuck Eye (Delmonico)

Best Cuts for Slow Cooking

Chuck Arm

Top Blade

Chuck Roast

Blade Chuck Roast

Bottom Round

Top Round

Best Cuts for the Oven

Chateaubriand

Shoulder Petite

Ribeye

Tri-tip

Top Sirloin Petite

Sirloin Tip

Cows provide a wealth of delicious and healthy animal proteins. While many forms such as milk and yogurt provide lactate, a natural sugar, when ingested with its natural fat and protein, it's somewhat mitigated. Plus cows deliver several other proteins and fats without lactate including butter, cheese and cream.

They provide large amounts of Leucine and Calcium and provide satiety.

Casein and Whey proteins are beneficial for both sustained and immediate energy, respectively. And both are readily absorbed when ingested in powder form.

POULTRY: THAT FIRST WHITE MEAT

Poultry is another versatile protein that is lower in saturated fat than beef and has earned its place as a lean alternative for those looking to shed some pounds. Often available in both white meat and dark meat varieties, they often allow for cuts with and without skin. And given its dense nutrition, it provides satiety. It's another protein that is difficult to ever-eat.

It has a rich nutrient offering including B vitamins, Selenium and Phosphorus.

White meat (breast and wings) provide more protein and less fat than their dark meat counterparts. But due to less saturated fat, it tends to be drier, and it's taste rather bland. It's perfect for blending in with any culinary style.

For every 100 grams of white chicken meat, 31 grams are protein, and only 4.6 grams are fat.

Dark Meat (legs and thighs) provide almost as much protein as white meat, but more fat, allowing for a juicier taste with a somewhat more distinctive taste.

For every 100 grams of dark chicken meat, 26 grams are protein, and 13.9 grams are fat. But they also provide higher amounts of Iron, Zinc and Niacin (B6).

If poultry is eaten with its skin, it adds extra calories and monounsaturated fats.

All cuts: Back, Breast, Leg, Thigh and Wing are well suited for grilling, stovetop, or roasting.

And then there's eggs. They are superior for muscle development because they contain all nine essential amino acids in the right ratio for human development—especially leucine. Eggs are easily digested and utilized throughout the body.

PORKY PIG, THAT OTHER WHITE MEAT

Pork is a versatile protein more popular in Asian cuisine, it still has an enviable reputation in the Western hemisphere. It's another protein that is available in both lean and fatty cuts, greatly impacting the taste and nutritional content.

It's high in Iron, Zinc, Selenium and Phosphorus and all the B vitamins as well as CLA.

Like Beef, it's great for cooking on the grill, stovetop or oven.

Best Cuts for Grilling
Pork Chops
Pork Tenderloin
Pork Ribs
Spareribs
Pork Sausage

Best Cuts for the Stovetop

Pork Chops

Pork Belly (braising)

Pork Shoulder (slow cooking)

Pork Butt

Spareribs

Pork Sausage

Bacon

Best Cuts for the Oven

Pork Chops

Pork Shoulder (slow cooking)

Pork Tenderloin

Pork Loin

Pork Leg

Spareribs

Pork Hock (slow cooking)

Ham (baking)

SILENCE OF THE BUFFALO, ELK AND DEER

Game meat is considered leaner and more nutrient dense than beef due to their active lives in the wild. Because these animals were range free when they were hunted, they were free of added hormones and antibiotics. However, they tend to have a gamier flavor that can be mitigated somewhat by certain precooking techniques such as aging the meat, marinating or using a dry rub.

Like pork, this meat is nutrient rich in Iron, Zinc, Selenium, Phosphorus and B vitamins. And their beneficial Omega 3 to Omega 6 ratio suggests that they may be supportive of hear health.

Bison in particular has lower cholesterol than traditional beef which may lead to better heart health. (In my opinion there is a great cholesterol debate in which this benefit would be moot.)

For every 100 grams of cooked bison, 28 grams are protein, while only 2.4 are fat.

For every 100 grams of cooked venison, 30 grams are protein, while only 3.2 grams are fat.

For every 100 grams of cooked elk, 26 grams are protein, while only 2.7 grams are fat.

Venison, Elk and Bison enjoy similar cuts as to those of beef for cooking.

FISHING FOR RELEVANCE

Both fish and shellfish deliver a host of nutritious options for fans of animal protein and rich sources of amino acids. Their abundance of Omega 3's is well documented, but salmon and tuna are especially good at building muscle. Both are highly digestible. But shrimp and other shellfish are also rich sources of selenium and zinc.

Four on the Podium: Tallow, Butter, Olive & Avocado Oil

These are pure fats. And even though Olive and Avocado oil come from fruits, their fat profile is superior to the plethora of vegetable oils that falsely tout their Omega 6 benefits. I use tallow for any grilling, frying or roasting that requires a high smoke point—around 400 degrees Fahrenheit. It gives a decadent flavor to poultry, shellfish, and lean meats. Butter is great for eggs and for acting as a finishing flavor for any beef. Be sure to look for grass fed varieties since regular butter can be loaded with added hormones and antibiotics.

When it comes to olive and avocado oils, they are utilized mainly as finishing oils or basics in dressings and sauces due to their lower smoke points. Unfortunately in both cases, the buyer should be aware of scams that could cost you money and your health. Olive Oil has become such a hot market, that the mafia has gotten involved in cutting them with cheap vegetable oils like Canola and smuggling them into the U.S. and other Western Countries. Given it prevalence, I have decided to only purchase those California grown and marked with a California Growers Association logo. The cartels have infiltrated the lucrative Avocado oil market as well, cutting most of those with cheap vegetable oils. I purchase Chosen brand as they have been shown to pass the oil purity test.

If you can't find either of these brands, try to find one that is sold in a dark glass bottle or metal tin. Also stick them in the fridge and see if they congeal. If they do, they're probably official. If they remain completely liquid, they're cut. Also the taste should be buttery and peppery and have a nice green tint. If it tastes bland or the color is off, chances are you bought a counterfeit batch.

It's All About the Animal Protein

Thanks for taking this quick health journey through the importance of animal protein in your diet. I hope raised some concerns with the Standard American Diet that is now making a lot of us sicker. By adopting at least a more Paleo approach to eating, you will find you feel better, have more energy and hopefully maintain your lean muscle mass if not add to it.

Changing a lifestyle is difficult. And if like most Americans, you find it difficult to give up on processed foods cold turkey, try a slower replacement approach where you add new animal proteins to your diet instead of cutting items out. As you increase the proteins you'll find that you're more satiated and can no longer eat everything. That's when you start to cut out the processed, manufactured foods.

Sources

Rd, J. K. M. (2023, April 24). *Vitamin A: benefits, deficiency, toxicity, and more.* Healthline. https://www.healthline.com/nutrition/vitamin-a

Rd, J. K. M. (2023b, August 7). *Essential amino acids: definition, benefits, and food sources.* Healthline. https://www.healthline.com/nutrition/essential-amino-acids

Rd, L. P. M. (2023, March 14). *What is thiamine deficiency? All you need to know.* Healthline. https://www.healthline.com/nutrition/thiamine-deficiency-symptoms

Rd, K. J. M. (2024, May 18). *4 Science-Based benefits of niacin (Vitamin B3).* Healthline. https://www.healthline.com/nutrition/niacin-benefits

Ld, L. S. M. R. (2018, October 1). *9 Health benefits of vitamin B6 (Pyridoxine).* Healthline. https://www.healthline.com/nutrition/vitamin-b6-benefits

Crider, C. (2023, November 6). *Vitamin B12: health benefits you may need to know about.* Healthline. https://www.healthline.com/health/vitamin-b12

Van De Walle Ms Rd, G. (2022, December 6). *5 Proven benefits of BCAAs (Branched-Chain amino Acids)*. Healthline. https://www.healthline.com/nutrition/benefits-of-bcaa

Rung, R. (2023, November 3). *How does calcium benefit your body and how much do you need?* Healthline. https://www.healthline.com/health/calcium

Superfoodly, & Superfoodly. (2021, February 18). *40 highest food sources of carnosine and benefits studied - SuperFoodly*. Superfoodly |. https://superfoodly.com/carnosine-benefits-and-natural-food-sources/

BSc, K. G. (2023, October 23). *CLA (Conjugated linoleic Acid): A detailed review*. Healthline. https://www.healthline.com/nutrition/conjugated-linoleic-acid

Cissn, R. M. M. (2023, November 2). *Everything you need to know about Creatine*. Healthline. https://www.healthline.com/nutrition/what-is-creatine

Rd, J. K. M. (2023a, March 16). *8 unique benefits of vitamin E*. Healthline. https://www.healthline.com/health/all-about-vitamin-e

Spritzler, F. (2023, June 28). *12 healthy foods that are high in iron*. Healthline. https://www.healthline.com/nutrition/healthy-iron-rich-foods

Ms, J. L. (2024, March 5). *Vitamin K2: Everything you need to know*. Healthline. https://www.healthline.com/nutrition/vitamin-k2

Ms, F. H. (2023, January 17). *17 Science-Based Benefits of omega-3 fatty acids.* Healthline. https://www.healthline.com/nutrition/17-health-ben efits-of-omega-3

Robertson, R., PhD. (2023, May 19). *Omega-3-6-9 fatty acids: A complete overview.* Healthline. https://www.healthline.com/nutrition/omega-3-6-9-overview

Clt, E. J. M. R. (2023, February 14). *Top 12 foods that are high in phosphorus.* Healthline. https://www.healthline.com/nutrition/foods-high-in-pho sphorus

Rd, J. K. M. (2023a, February 6). *7 Science-Based Health benefits of selenium.* Healthline. https://www.healthline.com/nutrition/selenium-benefits

Rd, J. K. M. (2022, November 28). *Zinc: Everything you need to know.* Healthline. https://www.healthline.com/nutrition/zinc

BEST BEEF CUTS FOR SLOW-COOKING. (2024). Beef Its What's for Dinner. Retrieved September 12, 2024, from https://www.beefitswhatsfordinne r.com/cuts/collection/33342/best-beef-cuts-for-slow-cooking

Best Beef Cuts for Oven Roasting. (2024). Beef It's What's for Dinner. Retrieved September 12, 2024, from https://www.beefitswhatsfordinne r.com/cuts/collection/33339/best-beef-cuts-for-oven-roasting

Leffler, S. (2023, November 28). *10 common pork cuts and the best way to cook with each of them.* Real Simple. https://www.realsimple.com/food-recipes/shopping-storing/food/common-cuts-pork

Watson, M. (2024, March 14). *A complete guide to pork cuts.* The Spruce Eats. https://www.thespruceeats.com/complete-guide-to-pork-cuts-4067791